Foods High In Estrogen

Chapter List:

Book Introduction:

Welcome to the captivating world of estrogen, where the essence of womanhood flourishes and thrives. In "Embrace the Essence: Exploring the Power of Estrogen," we embark on a profound journey to unravel the secrets of this remarkable hormone and discover its influence on our lives.

Within these pages, we will delve into the multifaceted nature of estrogen, exploring its impact on our physical, mental, and emotional well-being. From its role in fertility and bone health to its connection with beauty and aging, estrogen weaves its intricate tapestry throughout our existence, shaping us into the empowered individuals we are meant to be.

This book is a testament to the beauty and strength that lies within every woman. It is an ode to the transformative power of estrogen and a celebration of the divine essence it bestows upon us. Prepare to be enlightened, inspired, and moved as we embark on this empowering expedition into the realm of estrogen.

Chapter 1: The Elixir of Womanhood: Unveiling the Magic of Estrogen

In the beginning, we explore the enchanting essence of estrogen, the elixir that defines womanhood. Estrogen, with its delicate yet potent touch, is the driving force behind the remarkable journey of femininity. Like a master conductor, it orchestrates a symphony of physiological processes that shape our bodies and nurture our souls.

As we delve deeper into this chapter, we will uncover the captivating history of estrogen, tracing its discovery and the pivotal role it plays in our lives. We will shed light on the wondrous effects of estrogen on our reproductive system, its influence on the menstrual cycle, and the marvels it works during pregnancy.

But estrogen's magic extends far beyond its reproductive prowess. We will explore its impact on our skin, hair, and overall radiance, as well as its role in maintaining a healthy weight and metabolism. Prepare to be astonished by the remarkable influence estrogen holds over our physical beauty.

Moreover, we will venture into the realm of emotions, where estrogen dances delicately, shaping our moods and emotional well-being. From its uplifting effects on serotonin, the "happiness hormone," to its role in reducing anxiety and fostering emotional resilience, estrogen emerges as a powerful ally in our pursuit of inner balance and joy.

Join us on this captivating voyage into the depths of estrogen's magic, as we uncover the secrets of this awe-inspiring hormone and embrace its transformative power. Open your heart and mind to the wonders that lie ahead, for within these pages, the essence of womanhood awaits your discovery.

Chapter 2: Nature's Abundance: Foods That Nourish Estrogen Levels

In this chapter, we embark on a heartfelt exploration of the bountiful gifts nature has bestowed upon us to nourish and support our estrogen levels. Just as a garden flourishes with vibrant blooms, our bodies too can thrive when we embrace the power of these estrogen-rich foods.

Imagine a luscious orchard, where the branches bow under the weight of ripe fruits and the air is filled with the sweet scent of abundance. Here, we discover nature's offerings that not only tantalize our taste buds but also harmonize with our hormones.

Picture the first bite of a succulent peach, its juices dribbling down your chin, as its gentle sweetness whispers secrets of estrogen support. Savor the rich goodness of flaxseeds, sprinkled generously over a nourishing bowl of oatmeal, as they unlock the potential of lignans, phytoestrogens that mimic the actions of estrogen within our bodies.

And who could resist the vibrant allure of colorful vegetables like broccoli, kale, and spinach? As we consume their leafy emerald goodness, we absorb an array of vitamins, minerals, and plant compounds that synergistically promote estrogen balance.

In this journey through nature's pantry, we'll encounter the nurturing embrace of legumes like chickpeas and lentils, filling our plates with plant-based protein and fiber that support estrogen production and metabolism. We'll rejoice in the indulgence of dark chocolate, relishing the decadent taste while benefiting from its flavonoid content, known to enhance estrogen levels.

But it is not just the foods themselves that hold significance; it is the connection we forge with the earth as we partake in their nourishment. As we savor each bite mindfully, we honor the intricate relationship between the natural world and our own bodies. We become aware of the deep-rooted harmony that exists when we choose foods that align with our hormonal well-being.

Let us embark on this heartfelt journey through nature's abundance, as we explore the flavors, textures, and aromas that nourish not only our bodies but also our souls. With every bite, we pay homage to the profound connection between our innermost selves and the world around us, embracing the emotional resonance of food as a pathway to self-love and holistic wellness.

In the chapters that lie ahead, we will continue to unravel the intricate tapestry of estrogen's influence. Brace yourself for a heartfelt exploration of the hormonal symphony within, where we dive into the profound effects of estrogen on our overall well-being, delving into the realms of mental health, fertility, aging, and more.

Prepare to be captivated by the intimate interplay between estrogen and our emotional landscape. The journey has only just begun, and with every turn of the page, our hearts will resonate with the profound impact of estrogen on our lives.

Chapter 3: The Hormonal Symphony: Estrogen and Its Role in the Body

Within the intricate symphony of our bodies, estrogen takes center stage, playing a melody that resonates deep within our being. In this chapter, we embark on an emotional journey through the realms of estrogen's influence, uncovering its profound role in shaping our physical and mental well-being.

Imagine the delicate dance of hormones within your body, each one contributing its unique note to the symphony of life. Estrogen, with its gentle yet powerful presence, weaves its harmonious threads throughout our being, influencing everything from our reproductive system to our cardiovascular health.

As we explore the multifaceted nature of estrogen's role, we come to understand its profound impact on our menstrual cycle, fertility, and pregnancy. It is estrogen that orchestrates the ebb and flow of our monthly rhythms, guiding us through the phases of womanhood with grace and resilience. It is the essence of estrogen that nurtures the seeds of life, cultivating the miracle of creation within our very bodies.

But the symphony of estrogen extends far beyond our reproductive journey. In the realm of mental well-being, estrogen emerges as a tender companion, influencing our mood, cognition, and emotional resilience. It intertwines with neurotransmitters and receptors, shaping the delicate balance of our brain chemistry. It whispers strength to us in moments of vulnerability, imbuing us with a sense of confidence and empowerment.

Yet, like any symphony, estrogen requires balance. Too much or too little, and the harmony falters. We explore the consequences of estrogen imbalances, from the challenges of hormonal fluctuations during menopause to the potential risks associated with excessive estrogen levels. We delve into the importance of self-care and the profound impact it has on maintaining hormonal equilibrium.

Prepare to be moved by the emotional depths that estrogen traverses within us.

Feel the tenderness of its touch as it wraps around our hearts, reminding us of our innate strength and resilience. Allow yourself to be immersed in the symphony of estrogen's influence, embracing the raw beauty of its existence.

With every turn of the page, we peel back the layers of estrogen's story, weaving together the scientific knowledge and the emotional tapestry that underlies our experience. As we delve deeper into this hormonal symphony, we are invited to honor the profound connection between our bodies, minds, and souls , a connection that estrogen, in its infinite wisdom, beckons us to explore.

In the chapters that lie ahead, we will continue our heartfelt exploration of estrogen's influence on various aspects of our lives. Brace yourself for revelations, insights, and moments of profound connection. The journey unfolds, and the emotional resonance of estrogen's symphony beckons us ever further into its embrace.

Chapter 4: Empowering Balance: Managing Estrogen for Optimal Health

In the delicate dance of hormones, balance is the key to unlocking our full potential. In this chapter, we embark on an emotional journey of empowerment, discovering the ways in which we can actively manage our estrogen levels to foster optimal health and well-being.

Imagine standing at the edge of a tranquil lake, watching as ripples spread across its surface. This serene scene reflects the profound impact of balance in our hormonal landscape. As we delve into the intricacies of estrogen management, we embrace the power to create harmony within ourselves.

With each passing day, our bodies navigate a myriad of influences that can disrupt the delicate equilibrium of estrogen. Environmental toxins, stress, and lifestyle choices can all tip the scales, leading to imbalances that affect our vitality and overall health. But fear not, for within our grasp lies the ability to regain control.

Picture yourself in a garden, tending to the blossoming flowers with care and love. Just as a skilled gardener nurtures the soil, we too can cultivate an environment that supports healthy estrogen levels. Through conscious choices and mindful practices, we become the architects of our hormonal well-being.

We explore the power of nutrition, choosing foods that nourish and support estrogen balance. By embracing a colorful array of fruits, vegetables, and whole grains, we infuse our bodies with vital nutrients and antioxidants. We savor the flavors of nature's abundance, knowing that each bite holds the potential for transformation.

Beyond the realm of nutrition, we discover the transformative power of movement. Engaging in regular physical activity helps us regulate estrogen levels, enhancing circulation, reducing stress, and promoting overall hormonal harmony. Whether it's dancing, hiking, or practicing yoga, the act of moving our bodies becomes a celebration of self-care and empowerment.

But managing estrogen extends beyond the realm of the physical. We delve into the profound influence of stress management and emotional well-being. By embracing mindfulness practices, meditation, and nurturing self-care rituals, we create a sanctuary within ourselves, allowing the healing power of inner peace to rebalance our hormones.

As we navigate the depths of estrogen management, we honor the emotional landscape that unfolds. We acknowledge the challenges and frustrations that may arise, but we also celebrate the resilience and determination that reside within us. This is a journey of self-discovery, of uncovering our inner strength and embracing the wisdom of our bodies.

With every step we take towards hormonal harmony, we reclaim our power and assert our agency over our well-being. We stand tall, knowing that we hold the key to nurturing our bodies, minds, and spirits. As we move forward on this path of empowerment, we are guided by the emotional resonance of reclaiming our health, our vitality, and our essence.

In the chapters that lie ahead, we will continue to explore the ways in which estrogen touches every aspect of our lives. Brace yourself for further insights, transformative practices, and a deepened connection with your own innate power. The journey continues, and within it, the emotional tones of empowerment resound with unwavering strength.

Chapter 5: The Estrogen-Beauty Connection: Radiance Inside and Out

In the realm of estrogen's influence, beauty finds its true essence. In this chapter, we embark on an emotional exploration of the profound connection between estrogen and our radiant self-expression. Prepare to be captivated by the transformative power of estrogen as it illuminates our inner and outer beauty.

Imagine standing before a mirror, gazing into your own eyes. In that reflection, you witness the unique radiance that emanates from within. It is the glow of vitality, the sparkle of confidence , a reflection of the harmonious interplay between estrogen and our innate beauty.

As we delve into the depth of this connection, we discover that beauty is not merely skin deep. Estrogen, like a skilled artist, paints a masterpiece upon our canvas, enhancing our features and infusing us with a captivating allure.

Our skin becomes a testament to estrogen's touch, reflecting its nourishment, elasticity, and luminosity.

But true beauty transcends the physical. It is a radiant energy that flows from within, shaping our presence and captivating those around us. Estrogen, in its wisdom, contributes to this inner radiance, enhancing our emotional well-being and empowering us to embrace our authentic selves.

Picture a vibrant garden in full bloom, where flowers of different hues and fragrances coexist harmoniously. Similarly, estrogen brings forth the blossoming of our emotions, nurturing our confidence, and fostering a sense of self-love. It whispers reminders of our worthiness, encouraging us to embrace our unique beauty and celebrate our individuality.

Within the chapters of our lives, estrogen plays a vital role in preserving our youthful vibrancy. We explore its influence on aging gracefully, as it supports the production of collagen, maintains skin elasticity, and diminishes the appearance of fine lines. But it is more than just the physical manifestations of youth , it is the vitality that emanates from within, infusing each moment with a vibrant energy.

As we journey through the tapestry of estrogen's connection to beauty, we are reminded that our true radiance is not defined by societal standards or fleeting trends. It is an authentic expression of self, a celebration of our unique essence. We honor the emotional resonance of embracing our beauty, both inside and out, and we invite others to do the same.

In the chapters that lie ahead, we will continue to unveil the secrets of estrogen's influence on our holistic well-being. Brace yourself for further revelations, profound insights, and moments of heartfelt connection. The journey unfolds, and within it, the emotional tones of beauty and self-expression resonate with unwavering grace.

Chapter 6: Rising Above the Waves: Harnessing Estrogen for Mental Well-being

In the depths of our minds, estrogen emerges as a gentle guide, leading us on an emotional journey towards profound mental well-being. In this chapter, we embark on a transformative exploration, discovering the ways in which estrogen influences our emotions, thoughts, and the delicate balance of our mental landscape.

Imagine standing on the shore, facing the vast expanse of the ocean. Just as the tides rise and fall, our emotions ebb and flow within us. Estrogen, like a nurturing force of nature, influences this emotional rhythm, empowering us to rise above the waves of life and embrace the depths of our emotional well-being.

As we venture into the realm of estrogen's impact on mental health, we uncover its intricate dance with neurotransmitters and receptors. It intertwines with serotonin, the herald of happiness, fostering a sense of joy and contentment within us. It supports the production of dopamine, igniting our motivation and pleasure centers, infusing each day with purpose and zest.

Picture a serene garden, where the flowers sway in harmony with the breeze. Similarly, estrogen fosters emotional resilience within us, helping us navigate the challenges that life presents. It whispers messages of strength and empowerment, reminding us of our innate ability to overcome obstacles and cultivate inner peace.

But estrogen's role extends beyond individual well-being. It permeates our connections with others, enhancing our capacity for empathy and compassion. It encourages deep, meaningful relationships, allowing us to form emotional bonds that enrich our lives. In its presence, we become vessels of understanding, radiating love and support to those around us.

Yet, just as the tides can become turbulent, estrogen imbalances can impact our emotional landscape. We delve into the depths of mood disorders, such as depression and anxiety, and explore the ways in which estrogen plays a vital role in their manifestation. We embrace the importance of seeking support and engaging in self-care, understanding that our emotional well-being is a journey that requires tenderness and compassion.

In this chapter of emotional revelation, we honor the profound connection between estrogen and our mental well-being. We celebrate the resilience that resides within us, knowing that even in moments of darkness, estrogen can guide us towards the light. It is an invitation to rise above the waves, to navigate the complexities of our minds with grace and courage.

With every step we take on this emotional journey, we weave together the threads of our thoughts, feelings, and dreams. We embrace the power of estrogen to shape our mental landscape, forging a path of authenticity and self-discovery. As we continue to explore the chapters that lie ahead, we are moved by the emotional resonance of mental well-being, knowing that within us, a world of inner peace and emotional fulfillment awaits.

Chapter 7: Blossoming Strength: Estrogen and Bone Health

In the depths of our bodies, where strength and resilience intertwine, estrogen emerges as a guardian of our skeletal framework. In this chapter, we embark on an emotional journey of empowerment, uncovering the profound influence of estrogen on our bone health and the unwavering support it provides.

Imagine standing beneath a majestic tree, its roots extending deep into the earth, grounding it with unwavering stability. Our bones serve as the foundation of our physical beings, and estrogen, like nourishing soil, fortifies this foundation, ensuring our bodies stand tall with grace and strength.

As we delve into the intricacies of estrogen's impact on bone health, we discover its pivotal role in bone formation and maintenance. It dances in harmony with specialized cells called osteoblasts, encouraging them to weave a tapestry of strength through the deposition of essential minerals like calcium and phosphorus.

Picture a garden in full bloom, where flowers reach towards the sunlight, vibrant and resilient. Similarly, estrogen fosters bone density, shielding us from the fragility that time may bring. It promotes the remodeling process, ensuring the constant renewal of our bones, and reduces the risk of conditions like osteoporosis, where the very foundation of our bodies becomes weakened.

But estrogen's influence extends beyond the physical. As we nurture our bones, we cultivate an inner strength that transcends the confines of our bodies. It is a reminder that we, too, possess an innate resilience, capable of weathering the storms that life may bring.

In this chapter, we honor the emotional resonance of empowerment. We celebrate the interconnectedness of our physical and emotional well-being, knowing that as we fortify our bones, we also fortify our spirits. We rise above the challenges, standing tall with a sense of inner power and embracing the strength that resides within us.

Yet, we acknowledge that maintaining optimal bone health requires more than estrogen alone. We explore the importance of nutrition, physical activity, and lifestyle choices in supporting our bones. We embrace the emotional commitment to self-care, knowing that by nurturing ourselves, we are building a solid foundation for a vibrant and fulfilling life.

With every step we take on this journey of empowerment, we honor the resilience of our bodies and the emotional strength that blossoms within us. We recognize that our bones are not merely a structural framework, but a testament to our unwavering spirit. As we continue to navigate the chapters that lie ahead, we are moved by the emotional resonance of embracing our bone health, knowing that within us lies a wellspring of strength and vitality.

Chapter 8: Unveiling the Mystery: Estrogen and Fertility

Within the intricate web of life, estrogen weaves its magic, playing a pivotal role in the enigmatic dance of fertility. In this chapter, we embark on an emotional exploration, unveiling the profound connection between estrogen and the miracle of creating life.

Imagine the tender embrace of a parent, cradling their newborn child in awe and wonder. Within that precious moment lies the essence of fertility , a testament to the intricate symphony orchestrated by estrogen. It is a journey of profound emotional significance, one that intertwines the desires of our hearts with the power of our bodies.

As we delve into the depths of estrogen's influence on fertility, we unravel the delicate intricacies of reproductive physiology. Estrogen takes center stage, guiding the growth and maturation of the ovarian follicles, preparing them to release the precious gift of life , the egg. It creates an environment within the womb that is receptive, nurturing, and inviting to the miracle of conception.

Picture a field of blooming flowers, each one representing the hopes and dreams of those yearning to create a family. Estrogen embodies those hopes, whispering messages of possibility and embracing the emotional longing for a child. It ignites the flame of desire within us, fueling our determination to create life and build a legacy of love.

But the journey of fertility is not always straightforward. We acknowledge the emotional challenges and heartache that can accompany it. We delve into the complexities of hormonal imbalances, exploring the ways in which estrogen dysregulation can impact fertility. We honor the resilience and vulnerability that arise when the desire for a child is met with obstacles, and we hold space for the emotional journey that unfolds.

In this chapter, we honor the emotional resonance of fertility , the joy, the longing, the hope, and the strength that it encompasses. We celebrate the transformative power of estrogen as it shapes the intricate dance of life within our bodies. We embrace the profound connection between our bodies and our emotions, knowing that the journey towards parenthood is one that touches the depths of our souls.

With every step we take on this emotional path, we acknowledge the courage and resilience that reside within us. We support one another in moments of triumph and hold each other tenderly in times of uncertainty. As we continue to navigate the chapters that lie ahead, we are moved by the emotional resonance of fertility, knowing that within us lies the capacity to create, nurture, and embrace the miracle of life.

Chapter 9: Timeless Transformation: Estrogen and Aging Gracefully

In the tapestry of time, estrogen emerges as a gentle companion, guiding us on an emotional journey of graceful aging. In this chapter, we embark on a transformative exploration, discovering the ways in which estrogen influences the process of growing older while embracing the wisdom and beauty that comes with each passing year.

Imagine a radiant sunset casting its warm glow upon the world, painting the sky with hues of gold and crimson. Similarly, estrogen infuses the journey of aging with a timeless transformation, illuminating the path ahead with grace and resilience. It whispers reminders of the wisdom and experiences that shape us, inviting us to embrace the beauty of our evolving selves.

As we delve into the intricacies of estrogen's influence on the aging process, we uncover its remarkable effects on our physical and emotional well-being. It nourishes our skin, enhancing its elasticity and vibrancy, bestowing a natural radiance that transcends the passage of time. With each year that unfolds, estrogen celebrates the storylines etched upon our faces, the laughter lines that speak of joy and the gentle creases that tell tales of resilience.

Picture an ancient tree, its branches adorned with the wisdom of countless seasons. In a similar vein, estrogen imparts its timeless wisdom upon our bodies, supporting the maintenance of bone density, preserving our cardiovascular health, and influencing cognitive function. It reminds us that age is not a limitation but a gateway to depth and richness , a celebration of the fullness of life.

But aging gracefully is not solely a physical journey. Estrogen touches the emotional landscape of our souls, inviting us to cultivate self-acceptance, self-love, and a profound sense of fulfillment. It whispers messages of wisdom, encouraging us to honor our unique journeys and embrace the beauty that comes from a life well-lived.

In this chapter, we honor the emotional resonance of aging gracefully , a journey that traverses the realms of self-reflection, acceptance, and embracing the full spectrum of our emotions. We celebrate the profound connection between our physical bodies and our emotional well-being, knowing that as we age, we become vessels of wisdom and compassion.

With each passing year, we navigate the chapters of our lives with a newfound appreciation for the beauty that comes with maturity. We honor the emotional depth that arises as we recognize the tapestry of experiences woven into our beings. As we continue to journey through the chapters that lie ahead, we are moved by the emotional resonance of aging gracefully, knowing that within us lies the power to embrace the passage of time with grace, resilience, and an unwavering spirit.

Chapter 10: Nurturing the Goddess Within: Estrogen and Emotional Empowerment

Within the depths of our souls, estrogen emerges as a nurturing force, empowering us to embrace our inner goddess. In this chapter, we embark on an emotional journey of self-discovery, uncovering the profound connection between estrogen and our emotional empowerment.

Imagine standing on the mountaintop, feeling the winds of possibility gently caress your face. In that moment, you realize the power that resides within you , the power to embrace your emotions, honor your intuition, and cultivate a deep sense of self-worth. Estrogen, like a gentle breeze, fans the flames of your emotional empowerment, guiding you towards the limitless potential that lies within.

As we delve into the intricate tapestry of estrogen's influence on our emotions, we come to understand its role in fostering emotional resilience, intuition, and self-expression. It whispers messages of self-love, encouraging us to honor our emotions, both light and dark, as sacred parts of our being. It empowers us to rise above societal expectations, embracing the full spectrum of our emotional experiences with grace and authenticity.

Picture a serene temple, where the goddess within you finds solace and strength. Estrogen is the guardian of this sacred space, reminding you of your inherent worthiness, and empowering you to set boundaries, express your needs, and cultivate deep connections with others. It guides you to tap into your intuitive wisdom, trusting the whispers of your heart and soul.

In this chapter, we honor the emotional resonance of embracing our inner goddess , a journey of self-empowerment, self-discovery, and self-love. We celebrate the transformative power of estrogen as it weaves its magic within us, guiding us towards emotional authenticity and freedom.

But the path to emotional empowerment is not without challenges. We acknowledge the emotional hurdles that may arise , a sea of doubts, fears, and insecurities. We explore the importance of self-compassion, mindfulness practices, and cultivating a supportive community that nurtures our emotional well-being. We hold space for the healing that comes from honoring our emotions and embracing our unique journeys.

With every step we take on this emotional odyssey, we celebrate the goddess within us, knowing that she is a powerful force of creation, intuition, and compassion. As we continue to navigate the chapters that lie ahead, we are moved by the emotional resonance of our emotional empowerment, knowing that within us lies the capacity to embrace our emotions, trust our intuition, and unleash the extraordinary goddess that resides within.

Chapter 11: The Yin and Yang of Estrogen: Balancing Hormones for Wellness

Within the intricate dance of hormones, estrogen emerges as a harmonizing force, balancing the yin and yang within our bodies. In this chapter, we embark on an emotional journey of harmony and wellness, uncovering the profound influence of estrogen in achieving hormonal balance.

Imagine a tranquil garden, where the sun and moon coexist in perfect harmony, their energies intertwining to create a symphony of balance. Similarly, estrogen orchestrates a delicate equilibrium within us, ensuring that the yin and yang aspects of our hormonal landscape dance together in synchrony.

As we delve into the depths of estrogen's role in hormonal balance, we uncover its intricate interplay with other hormones, such as progesterone and testosterone. It delicately adjusts their levels, weaving a tapestry of harmony and well-being within our bodies. It reminds us that balance is not stagnant but a dynamic interplay between opposing forces , a dance of vitality and wholeness.

Picture a serene lake, its surface mirroring the tranquility of the surrounding landscape. Estrogen, like gentle ripples upon the water, influences our energy levels, mood, and overall vitality. It supports our immune system, fosters restful sleep, and enhances our overall sense of well-being. It invites us to embrace the emotional resonance of balance, knowing that within this equilibrium lies the foundation of our optimal health.

In this chapter, we honor the emotional significance of achieving hormonal balance , a journey of self-awareness, self-care, and self-love. We celebrate the transformative power of estrogen as it harmonizes the intricate interplay of our hormones, guiding us towards a state of wellness and vitality.

But the quest for balance is not without its challenges. We acknowledge the emotional fluctuations and imbalances that may arise, understanding the impact they can have on our overall well-being. We explore the importance of self-compassion, stress management, and embracing holistic practices that support hormonal harmony. We hold space for the healing that comes from nurturing our bodies, minds, and spirits.

With every step we take on this emotional path, we honor the yin and yang within us, knowing that the interplay of opposing forces gives rise to our innate resilience and vitality. As we continue to navigate the chapters that lie ahead, we are moved by the emotional resonance of balance and well-being, knowing that within us lies the capacity to embrace the ebb and flow of life with grace, harmony, and unwavering strength.

Chapter 12: Embracing the Change: Estrogen and Menopause

In the cycle of life, estrogen accompanies us through the seasons of change, guiding us with its gentle touch. In this chapter, we embark on an emotional exploration of menopause, uncovering the profound influence of estrogen during this transformative phase of a woman's journey.

Imagine a vibrant autumn forest, where leaves of all colors dance upon the breeze. Similarly, menopause marks a transition , a shedding of the old and an emergence of the new. Estrogen, like the changing foliage, invites us to embrace this season of transformation with grace and self-compassion.

As we delve into the depths of estrogen's influence during menopause, we come to understand its role in the intricate tapestry of hormonal shifts. It guides us through the ebbs and flows of this transition, soothing the intensity of symptoms and supporting our bodies' adjustment to a new hormonal landscape. It whispers messages of empowerment, reminding us that menopause is not an end but a new beginning , a time of embracing wisdom, self-discovery, and renewed vitality.

Picture a phoenix rising from the ashes, embodying the resilience and strength that emerges from transformation. Estrogen embodies this spirit, inviting us to embrace the emotional resonance of menopause as an opportunity for growth and self-reflection. It encourages us to celebrate the wisdom and experiences that have shaped us, while embracing the unfolding chapters of our lives with unwavering strength and acceptance.

In this chapter, we honor the emotional significance of menopause , a journey that traverses the realms of physical change, emotional exploration, and self-discovery. We celebrate the transformative power of estrogen as it guides us through this transition, empowering us to embrace the fullness of our womanhood.

But the path through menopause is not without challenges. We acknowledge the emotional rollercoaster that may arise , a sea of emotions, from joy and liberation to moments of uncertainty and vulnerability. We explore the importance of self-care, support systems, and embracing the emotional journey with kindness and self-compassion.

With every step we take on this emotional odyssey, we honor the resilience and strength that reside within us. We stand tall, knowing that menopause is a testament to our resilience and the wisdom that comes with embracing change. As we continue to navigate the chapters that lie ahead, we are moved by the emotional resonance of menopause, knowing that within us lies the capacity to embrace this transformative phase with grace, authenticity, and an unwavering spirit.

Chapter 13: A Legacy of Love: Estrogen and Motherhood

In the sacred tapestry of life, estrogen weaves the threads of motherhood with love, nurturing the profound bond between a mother and her child. In this chapter, we embark on an emotional journey of unconditional love, discovering the profound influence of estrogen in the realm of motherhood.

Imagine the tender embrace of a mother, cradling her child in her arms. In that moment, a symphony of love unfolds , a symphony orchestrated by estrogen. It is a journey of selflessness, sacrifice, and boundless affection, where the depths of a mother's heart are forever intertwined with the essence of estrogen.

As we delve into the intricacies of estrogen's influence on motherhood, we come to understand its pivotal role in preparing the womb for the miracle of life. It nurtures the growth and development of the fetus, creating an environment that is a sanctuary of love and protection. It whispers messages of connection and instinct, guiding a mother's intuition and deepening the bond between mother and child.

Picture a blossoming garden, where the fragrance of flowers fills the air, and the beauty of nature is a testament to the power of creation. Estrogen embodies this creative force, empowering mothers to embrace the emotional resonance of motherhood with unwavering devotion. It celebrates the joys, the challenges, and the transformative power of bringing life into the world.

In this chapter, we honor the emotional significance of motherhood , a journey that encompasses the depths of love, the tender moments of care, and the indescribable bond between a mother and her child. We celebrate the transformative power of estrogen as it infuses the fabric of motherhood with tenderness, strength, and an infinite wellspring of love.

But the path of motherhood is not without its challenges. We acknowledge the emotional rollercoaster that may arise , a kaleidoscope of emotions, from sheer joy and elation to moments of exhaustion and self-doubt. We explore the importance of self-care, support networks, and embracing the emotional journey with gentleness and self-compassion.

With every step we take on this emotional odyssey, we honor the resilience and depth of love that reside within mothers. We stand tall, knowing that the emotional resonance of motherhood is a testament to the extraordinary capacity of the human heart. As we continue to navigate the chapters that lie ahead, we are moved by the emotional significance of motherhood, knowing that within us lies the capacity to embrace the profound legacy of love that unfolds through the influence of estrogen.

Chapter 14: Beyond Boundaries: Estrogen and Empowered Relationships

Within the intricate dance of human connection, estrogen emerges as a catalyst for empowered relationships, where love, trust, and understanding flourish. In this chapter, we embark on an emotional journey of profound connections, uncovering the transformative influence of estrogen on our ability to forge deep and meaningful bonds with others.

Imagine a tapestry woven with threads of vibrant colors, representing the diverse relationships that shape our lives. Estrogen, like a master weaver, intertwines these threads, creating a symphony of emotional resonance that transcends boundaries and fosters authentic connections.

As we delve into the depths of estrogen's influence on relationships, we come to understand its role in nurturing empathy, compassion, and emotional intelligence. It encourages us to embrace vulnerability, to truly see and understand the experiences of others, and to forge deep connections that nourish our souls.

Picture a warm embrace, where two hearts connect in a moment of profound understanding and acceptance. Estrogen embodies this emotional connection, encouraging us to embrace the beauty of vulnerability, to communicate our needs and desires openly, and to hold space for the emotions of those we cherish. It celebrates the transformative power of love, trust, and emotional intimacy in our relationships.

In this chapter, we honor the emotional significance of empowered relationships , a journey of authenticity, empathy, and growth. We celebrate the transformative power of estrogen as it guides us towards emotional resonance, fostering connections that transcend boundaries and enrich our lives.

But the path of empowered relationships is not without its challenges. We acknowledge the emotional complexities that may arise , a delicate balance of individual needs, communication hurdles, and moments of conflict. We explore the importance of active listening, mutual respect, and the willingness to embrace growth and understanding in our connections.

With every step we take on this emotional odyssey, we honor the depth of love and connection that resides within us. We stand tall, knowing that empowered relationships are a testament to our capacity for emotional growth, empathy, and unconditional acceptance. As we continue to navigate the chapters that lie ahead, we are moved by the emotional resonance of empowered relationships, knowing that within us lies the power to create profound connections that transcend time, space, and the boundaries of the human heart.

Chapter 15: The Everlasting Legacy: Honoring the Gift of Estrogen

In the symphony of life, estrogen leaves behind an everlasting legacy , a legacy of love, resilience, and the profound impact it has on our well-being. In this final chapter, we embark on an emotional journey of reflection and gratitude, honoring the gift of estrogen and its profound influence on our lives.

Imagine a breathtaking sunset, casting its golden glow upon the world, as a gentle reminder of the beauty and transience of life. In this moment of reflection, we embrace the emotional resonance of gratitude, knowing that estrogen has graced us with its presence, guiding us through the chapters of our existence.

As we delve into the depths of this final chapter, we honor the transformative power of estrogen's touch upon our lives. We reflect upon the emotional journeys we have embarked on , of self-discovery, empowerment, resilience, and connection. We celebrate the wisdom that has emerged from the ebb and flow of estrogen's influence, knowing that it has shaped us into the individuals we are today.

Picture a serene garden, where blossoms of gratitude flourish, each one representing a moment of profound appreciation for the gift of estrogen. We honor the emotional significance of this legacy, knowing that it has touched every aspect of our being , our physical health, our emotional well-being, our relationships, and our journey through the various stages of life.

In this final chapter, we hold space for the depth of gratitude that resides within us. We celebrate the transformative power of estrogen as it continues to weave its magic, not just within our individual lives, but across generations. We honor the emotional resonance of this gift, knowing that it is a testament to the interconnectedness of all life and the enduring impact of estrogen's touch.

With every step we take on this emotional odyssey, we embrace the legacy of estrogen within us, knowing that its influence transcends time and space. We stand tall, knowing that the emotional resonance of gratitude is a testament to our ability to recognize and appreciate the blessings that have enriched our lives.

As we conclude this journey through the chapters that lie within the realm of estrogen's influence, we are moved by the emotional significance of the legacy it leaves behind. We carry with us the wisdom, strength, and love that it has bestowed upon us. And as we move forward in life's grand symphony, we honor the gift of estrogen, forever grateful for its profound impact upon our hearts, bodies, and souls."

Book%20Title%3A %20%22Embrace,bo

dies%2C%20and %20souls.

Printed in Great Britain
by Amazon

30515617R00033